WASTE

The Environmental Crisis and the Urgent Need for Change

AMANDA PLAISTED

Copyright © 2023 by Amanda Plaisted

Contents

Introduction: The State of Our Environment

There was a little girl named Maya, she was a keen and attentive youngster who was always interested in what was going on around her. She became more aware of something unsettling as she grew older: the atmosphere around her was changing, and not for the better.

The once-beautiful woodland on her town's outskirts was gradually disappearing, replaced by huge houses and concrete. The river that formerly ran through her hamlet has become dark and dirty, with debris floating on its surface.

The fog in the air made it difficult for her to take a deep breath.

Maya decided one day that she couldn't stand by and watch her beautiful land be destroyed. She encouraged her classmates and friends to join the "Green Earth Club," an organization committed to fighting the environmental disaster they were experiencing.

They organized clean-up drives in their local parks and beaches, clearing up garbage. They began a recycling program at their school, encouraging students to decrease waste and repurpose items. They planted trees and flowers in bleak locations, restoring life and color to the formerly lonely landscapes.

People in the neighborhood took notice as their initiatives gained traction. Maya and her friends spread the word about the significance of living a sustainable lifestyle through lectures, seminars, and community activities. They encouraged their parents and neighbors to make minor changes in their everyday lives, such as using reusable bags and bottles, conserving electricity, and supporting environmentally friendly companies.

As word of their amazing efforts spread, additional towns and cities quickly joined their cause. Communities banded together to address the environmental disaster, and the movement spread quickly. It didn't take long for governments and companies to recognize the urgency of the situation as well.

Maya and her friends were asked to speak at worldwide conferences, where they shared their firsthand experiences and inspired others to act. They worked with scientists, engineers, and specialists from numerous sectors to discover creative solutions to urgent concerns such as pollution, deforestation, and climate change.

Maya's and the Green Earth Club's efforts made a noticeable effect over time. The air grew fresher, the river began to run crystal clear again, and animals returned to formerly desolate places. Their village became a model of sustainable living, spurring reform throughout the country.

But the labor was far from done. Maya understood that maintaining a healthy atmosphere demanded constant work and awareness. She made it her job to teach future generations about the value of maintaining and safeguarding the Earth they inherited.

Maya grew up to become a renowned environmental activist and dedicated her life to making the world a more sustainable and harmonious place. Her influence echoed through the generations, leaving a legacy of optimism, resilience, and a renewed feeling of responsibility for the environment.

As a result, Maya and the Green Earth Club's narrative serves as a reminder that every one of us can affect change. It is a call to action, pushing us to stand up for the environment and become environmental stewards. We can convert the current condition of our environment into one of restoration, rejuvenation, and plenty for all living species by working together. In a world where development is frequently at the expense of the environment, our planet is at a crucial juncture. As human civilization has grown, so has our influence on nature's fragile equilibrium. From enormous concrete jungles encroaching on once-pristine landscapes to black clouds of pollution obscuring the skies, evidence of our disdain for the environment can be seen everywhere.

Oceans, which were once teeming with life and dynamic ecosystems, are today plagued by plastic pollution, overfishing, and coral reef bleaching. Landscapes that were previously brimming with varied flora and animals are being devastated at an alarming rate to make way for industrial expansion and resource exploitation. And, as global energy demand rises, we continue to burn fossil fuels, spewing greenhouse gasses into the atmosphere and contributing to the worrisome rise in global temperatures.

The repercussions of our choices are not a distant danger; they are a present reality. Extreme weather events, melting ice caps, and rising sea levels serve as harsh reminders of the urgency with which the environmental crisis must be addressed. Ecosystems are disintegrating, biodiversity is dwindling, and our very life is threatened.

However, this is not a depressing narrative, but rather a call to action. Individuals and communities all across the world are standing up to take on the duty of protecting and restoring our environment. Scientists, activists, and ordinary residents are banding together to promote sustainable practices, renewable energy, and conservation measures.

Technological advancements provide promise for a greener future. Renewable energy sources including solar, wind, and hydroelectric electricity are becoming increasingly accessible and cost-effective. Electric vehicles are becoming more popular, reducing our reliance on fossil fuels and lowering hazardous pollutants. Sustainable agricultural methods are being developed to decrease soil degradation, increase biodiversity, and limit the use of toxic chemicals.

Education and awareness are critical for effecting change. Environmental studies are being integrated into school and university curricula, educating the future generation on the necessity of maintaining our world. Environmental groups and grassroots movements raise awareness through campaigns, social media, and community participation, pushing people to adopt environmentally responsible decisions in their everyday lives.

However, time is important. To ameliorate the environmental disaster and protect our planet's future, we must act quickly and forcefully. Governments, businesses, and people must all embrace sustainable practices, prioritize conservation efforts, and become change agents. We can mend the scars on our environment by working together to establish a future in which humans and nature dwell in peace.

The status of our ecosystem is in jeopardy, but we can alter the tide. Let this book serve as a reminder that our choices today will determine the fate of our world. Let us all pledge to become Earth stewards, working toward a future in which our environment is one of vibrant ecosystems, clean air and water, and a sustainable balance between human development and the natural world.

Chapter 1. The Evolution of Waste: From Ancient Times to the Present

Human civilization has always produced waste in many kinds. The way cultures dealt with trash has changed dramatically from ancient times to the present. This chapter will present a brief history of trash management and disposal.

Civilizations of Antiquity

Waste management was quite straightforward in ancient times. The majority of garbage was organic, such as food scraps, and was permitted to degrade naturally. This organic waste was frequently used as agricultural fertilizer. However, as civilizations advanced and became more urbanized, waste management became a more serious concern.

The Roman Empire and the Middle Ages

Several cities had trash collecting systems throughout the Roman Empire. The Romans developed complex subterranean sewage systems to remove garbage and rain, therefore improving sanitary standards. Cities in medieval Europe often had dedicated garbage disposal places outside the walls, which often resulted in unclean living conditions. Waste was occasionally poured into rivers, contaminating them and spreading illness.

The Great Industrial Revolution

During the 18th and 19th centuries, the rise of industrialization created substantial environmental issues. Massive volumes of garbage were created as a result of rapid urbanization and industrial activities. Waste, especially harmful industrial wastes, was frequently thrown into surrounding bodies of water, contaminating the ecosystem further. In certain cities, this time also witnessed the beginnings of systematic trash collection and disposal systems. In the late 18th century, for example, London created a private rubbish collection service, collecting and transporting waste to specified disposal locations.

The Rise of Landfills in the 20th Century

Waste management strategies advanced during the twentieth century. In many nations, landfills have become the principal method of garbage disposal. To reduce odor and vermin, waste was deposited in big designated areas and covered with layers of dirt. However, a lack of effective waste segregation and hazardous material disposal raised environmental issues. The introduction of plastics and the subsequent throwaway culture in the mid-twentieth century created new waste management difficulties. The inappropriate disposal of plastic garbage caused massive contamination in the seas and landfills. Recycling and garbage reduction projects began to gain pace, to reduce waste's environmental effects.

Modern Times and Eco-Friendly Practices

Waste management has become a serious worldwide concern in recent decades. Many governments have introduced waste-reduction methods, such as encouraging recycling, composting, and waste-to-energy technology. Recycling programs have grown to embrace a wider range of materials, as have attempts to educate the public about trash separation and its environmental effect. Furthermore, the circular economy concept has gained traction as a sustainable waste management strategy. The goal is to create a closed-loop system by reusing, repurposing, and recycling resources to reduce waste creation. This shift focuses on lowering resource usage and maximizing product lifecycle, hence reducing overall waste generation.

Advances in waste-to-energy technologies such as incineration and anaerobic digestion have enabled an alternate method of trash disposal while also producing electricity. These procedures contribute to the

reduction of landfill trash
and the use of renewable
energy sources.

Waste management is
evolving as we move deeper
into the twenty-first
century. The emphasis on
sustainable practices,
technology breakthroughs,
and public awareness of
garbage's environmental
impact all contribute to
continuous improvements in
waste management systems
across the world.

Throughout history, waste
management has seen
tremendous modifications.
From ancient civilizations to
the present day,
communities have
constantly adapted and
evolved strategies to
manage the rising issue of
garbage disposal. While
previous approaches
frequently had severe
environmental implications,
the present period supports
sustainable waste
management strategies to
reduce environmental

impact and transition to a more circular and efficient system.

Chapter 2. Impact of Waste on Ecosystems: Destruction and Degradation

Throughout history, poor waste/garbage disposal and management techniques have wreaked havoc on our natural world. Waste has had far-reaching impacts on the delicate balance of ecosystems, from polluting water bodies to contaminating soils.The influence of garbage on ecosystems is particularly obvious in maritime habitats. Plastic trash, such as bottles, bags, and fishing gear, has resulted in the creation of massive garbage patches in the world's oceans. These floating garbage islands not only endanger marine life but also emit hazardous chemicals as they degrade, contaminating the water and compromising the health of aquatic ecosystems. Seabirds, turtles, and marine mammals, among others, might become entangled in the trash or mistake it for food, resulting in damage or death.

Similarly, industrial and residential trash poisoning of water bodies has disastrous consequences on freshwater ecosystems. Chemical pollutants and harmful compounds from inappropriate waste disposal wind up in lakes, rivers, and streams, polluting the water and harming aquatic creatures' health. The unregulated discharge of oil and toxic chemicals has resulted in disastrous mishaps, such as oil spills, which have ravaged marine ecosystems and had long-term ecological implications. Waste has a big influence on terrestrial ecosystems as well. Inadequately managed landfills can pollute soils and groundwater with dangerous compounds such as heavy metals, pesticides, and garbage leachate. These toxins can last for years in the ecosystem and permeate into nearby places, damaging plant and animal life. Furthermore, organic waste disposal in landfills emits methane, a strong greenhouse gas that contributes to climate change and further damages ecosystems.

Deforestation, which is caused in part by increased garbage output and the demand for landfills, also contributes to ecosystem deterioration. Forests are frequently removed to make way for trash disposal sites, resulting in the loss of critical ecosystems and a decrease in biodiversity.

Furthermore, garbage incineration generates pollutants and releases toxic gasses into the environment, contributing to air pollution and respiratory difficulties in humans and animals alike.

Waste has an influence on ecosystems that extends beyond the surrounding environment. The deterioration of ecosystems affects natural processes that are essential for the health and survival of all living creatures, such as nutrient cycling and pollination. These disturbances can have a domino effect, resulting in the extinction of plant and animal species, habitat loss, and an imbalance in ecological relationships.

Managing the impact of trash on ecosystems necessitates a multifaceted strategy. It all starts with lowering waste output through sustainable activities like recycling, reusing, and embracing a circular economy perspective. Waste management systems must be created and updated to guarantee appropriate waste disposal and treatment while reducing environmental consequences. Education and awareness efforts are critical in encouraging people and communities to practice appropriate trash disposal.

Furthermore, the development and deployment of eco-friendly technology, such as improved recycling and garbage treatment facilities, may greatly minimize trash's environmental effects. Governments and organizations have a critical role in developing and implementing waste management legislation to guarantee accountability and environmental protection.

Chapter 3. The Health Effects of Waste: From Air Pollution to Contaminated Water

The quantity of garbage produced, from industrial to municipal, is expanding at an alarming rate. Waste not only causes environmental problems, but it also has serious health consequences for individuals.

Air pollution is one of the health repercussions of trash. When garbage is burnt, hazardous gasses and particles are released into the sky. These contaminants have been linked to asthma, bronchitis, and possibly lung cancer. Prolonged exposure to waste-related air pollution can potentially contribute to heart disease

and other cardiovascular problems.
When it comes to garbage, another health risk is contaminated water. Improper trash disposal can damage water supplies, rendering them hazardous for human consumption. People who drink polluted water are in danger of contracting waterborne illnesses such as cholera, dysentery, and hepatitis. These illnesses can cause severe diarrhea, vomiting, dehydration, and even death in certain cases.
Pests such as rodents, flies, and mosquitoes are also drawn to waste. These pests are disease carriers and can transmit them to people. Rats, for example, are recognized carriers of illnesses such as leptospirosis and hantavirus, whereas mosquitos are known carriers of malaria, dengue fever, and Zika Virus. These disorders can cause a variety

of symptoms, ranging from a little discomfort to life-threatening problems.

Furthermore, garbage has the potential to pollute soil and agricultural output. When garbage is improperly disposed of near agricultural regions, the soil can get polluted with hazardous chemicals and diseases. As a result, crops and food cultivated in these locations may absorb these toxins, rendering them unfit for human consumption. Consuming contaminated food can cause food poisoning, gastrointestinal disorders, and possibly long-term health concerns.

Finally, trash may have an emotional impact on individuals and society. Living in high-waste regions can induce tension, worry, and feelings of powerlessness. The sight and smell of trash can be unpleasant, contributing to a low quality of life. Furthermore, being aware of the health dangers involved with trash might have a detrimental influence on mental health.

Proper waste management is critical for mitigating the health impacts of trash. Implementing successful recycling and trash reduction initiatives, as well as suitable disposal procedures that limit environmental pollution, are all part of this. Communities and governments should collaborate to educate people about the importance of trash management and to encourage proper garbage disposal methods.

Furthermore, standards and regulations must be implemented to enforce effective waste management methods. This involves monitoring and regulating companies to ensure that waste management requirements are followed. Implementing higher emission limits for industry and promoting clean technology can also assist minimize waste-related air pollution.

Furthermore, increasing access to safe drinking water is critical in the prevention of waterborne illnesses caused by waste pollution. Investing in water treatment facilities and educating people about clean water practices can help safeguard communities from the detrimental consequences of waste.

Overall, addressing the health implications of garbage necessitates a multifaceted strategy that considers both the environment and public health. We can reduce the health hazards connected with garbage by emphasizing effective waste management and implementing sustainable practices, resulting in a better and safer environment for everyone.

Chapter 4. Landfills and Waste Management: Current Practices and Challenges

Landfills and garbage management are critical components in dealing with the massive quantity of waste created by human activity. However, existing waste management techniques and problems offer substantial environmental and public health risks. Landfills are constructed to bury and store garbage, therefore serving as a regulated disposal location. They are frequently used as the principal method of trash disposal across the world, however, their environmental effect may be significant. One of the most serious problems linked with landfills is the release of greenhouse gasses, notably methane. Methane is released into the atmosphere when garbage decomposes, contributing to global warming and climate change.

Furthermore, the physical structure of landfills poses difficulties. Toxic chemicals and toxins from garbage can leach into soil and groundwater, endangering neighboring ecosystems and even poisoning water supplies. If not adequately handled and cleaned, leachate, a liquid byproduct created as garbage decomposes, can constitute a serious concern.

Another major issue is the continuous upkeep and management of landfills. Proper monitoring and control techniques are essential for preventing uncontrollable fires, odor problems, and insect infestations. Landfills, if not managed properly, can become breeding grounds for disease-carrying insects and vermin, posing serious health threats to adjacent people.

Aside from these difficulties, land scarcity is becoming a growing concern, particularly in metropolitan areas. Finding adequate space for new landfills is becoming increasingly difficult, complicating waste management solutions. Because of this constraint, alternate waste management systems such as recycling, composting, and waste-to-energy technologies have become necessary.

Several techniques might be taken to alleviate the present issues related to landfills and waste management. To begin, a change toward trash reduction and recycling at the source is required. Promoting trash management awareness and education, as well as encouraging individuals and organizations to minimize waste generation and improve recycling efforts, may have a substantial influence.

Additionally, landfill design and construction may be improved to reduce environmental problems. Liners are used in modern landfills to keep leachate from polluting groundwater, and gas collection systems are used to catch methane and transform it into electricity. Regular monitoring and maintenance of landfills are also required to maintain effective operation and risk mitigation.

Another crucial component is to investigate alternate waste management systems. Organic waste, such as food scraps and yard trimmings, may be composted to decrease landfill trash while also providing important nutrient-rich compost. garbage-to-energy systems such as incineration and anaerobic digestion may extract energy from garbage while lowering methane emissions.

Collaboration between government, industry, and communities is critical in solving landfill and waste management concerns. Governments can establish stronger rules and policies to encourage sustainable waste management practices while also incentivizing recycling and trash reduction. Industries must invest in cleaner technology and use sustainable procedures to reduce waste output. Communities may take an active role by educating themselves, adopting safe garbage disposal, and supporting local recycling efforts.

Chapter 5. Plastic Pollution: The Silent Killer of our Oceans

Plastic pollution has emerged as one of the most important environmental concerns of our day, particularly in our seas. Plastic garbage poured into seas and streams has disastrous repercussions for marine life and ecosystem health. Plastic pollution is frequently referred to as our oceans' silent killer, causing devastation beneath the surface.

Plastic trash in our seas is astounding, ranging from plastic bottles and bags to microplastics. Over 8 million tons of plastic trash are anticipated to reach the seas each year. This garbage not only endangers marine species physically, but it also releases hazardous chemicals and pollutants into the sea.

Plastic trash is sometimes mistaken for food by marine species, resulting in disastrous effects. Sea turtles, for example, have been observed ingesting plastic bags, mistaking them for jellyfish. These sacks can clog their digestive systems, resulting in delayed and agonizing deaths. Plastic ingestion or entanglement also causes injury, malnutrition, and asphyxia in seabirds, dolphins, seals, and whales.

Microplastics, which are little plastic particles smaller than 5mm in size, are considerably more dangerous. They are produced by the decomposition of bigger plastic trash or are purposefully incorporated into goods such as cosmetics and exfoliating scrubs. Because microplastics are frequently too tiny to be cleaned out by water treatment facilities, they wind up in our seas. Microplastics are mistaken for food by marine species such as fish and shellfish, potentially leading to the transmission of these pollutants up the food chain and eventually to people who consume seafood.

Plastic pollution has an impact that extends beyond damaging marine life. It also destabilizes ecosystems and harms crucial coastal habitats. Coral reefs, for example, are becoming increasingly endangered as plastic garbage suffocates them, limiting the passage of oxygen and nutrients and eventually leading to their demise. To address the issue of plastic pollution, a multifaceted strategy is required. Education and awareness efforts are critical in teaching the public about the risks of plastic trash as well as encouraging appropriate consumption and waste management methods. Individuals may limit their plastic footprint by using reusable bags, bottles, and utensils and recycling or disposing of plastic garbage responsibly.

To prevent plastic pollution, legislation, and policy reforms are also required. Governments must pass and implement single-use plastic bans, encourage producer accountability, and invest in recycling infrastructure. Companies should be accountable for the complete lifespan of their products, including package collection and recycling, under extended producer responsibility.

Plastic pollution may be reduced by innovation and research into alternative materials and packaging solutions. Alternatives to single-use plastics include biodegradable and compostable materials, as well as sustainable packaging choices.

Furthermore, advances in waste management technology, such as enhanced recycling procedures and waste-to-energy systems, can help reduce the quantity of plastic garbage that ends up in our seas.

We must act immediately to address the plastic pollution catastrophe in our seas. We can minimize plastic trash, safeguard marine life, and conserve the health and biodiversity of our oceans via joint efforts and worldwide collaboration. Every action we take, no matter how little, can contribute to a cleaner, healthier future for our seas and future generations.

Chapter 6.
Chemical and Toxin Dangers in Industrial Waste

Concerns about the risks of industrial waste and its influence on the environment and human health have grown in recent years. Byproducts and pollutants created by industrial operations, such as chemicals, poisons, and hazardous materials, are referred to as industrial waste.

Pollution of the air, water, and soil is one of the biggest hazards linked with industrial waste. When these wastes are inappropriately disposed of or released into the environment, they have the potential to pollute vital resources on which humans and ecosystems rely. This pollution has the potential to harm both the environment and human health.

Toxins and chemicals found in industrial waste can pollute water supplies, making them hazardous for drinking, fishing, and irrigation. When polluted water sources are ingested or utilized for agricultural reasons, they can cause a variety of health difficulties, including gastrointestinal ailments, reproductive troubles, and even cancer. Polluted water may also be harmful to aquatic life, resulting in the death of fish and other aquatic species.

Another big threat posed by industrial waste is air pollution. Pollutants released into the atmosphere, such as greenhouse gasses, particulate matter, and volatile organic compounds, can contribute to global warming, climate change, and respiratory issues in people. Inhaling these contaminants can cause respiratory disorders including asthma, bronchitis, and lung cancer. Furthermore, airborne pollutants can have long-term consequences on human health, such as neurological diseases and developmental concerns. Furthermore, industrial waste may pollute soil, rendering it unsuited for cultivation and endangering food safety. Toxins can infiltrate the food chain and eventually wind up in the human population when crops and plants absorb them, creating a variety of health concerns.

To mitigate the hazards of industrial waste, industries must use sustainable waste management techniques. This involves actions such as recycling, waste minimization, and the adoption of cleaner manufacturing practices. Waste materials must also be properly treated and disposed of to be released into the environment as little as possible.

The role of governments in regulating and enforcing waste management policies is critical. They must implement and enforce rigorous legislation to guarantee that the industry handles their garbage correctly. Furthermore, public education and knowledge about the risks of industrial waste are critical in encouraging citizens and communities to demand cleaner practices and hold businesses accountable for their activities.

Industrial waste endangers both the environment and human health. Toxins and chemicals released into the air, water, and soil can have disastrous consequences for ecosystems, animals, and human populations. Industry must embrace sustainable waste management procedures, and governments must enforce legislation and raise public awareness. Only by working together can we reduce the hazards of industrial waste and ensure a better and safer environment for future generations.

Chapter 7. The Role of Consumerism: How Our Decisions Contribute to Waste

Consumerism, without a doubt, contributes significantly to waste in our society. We are continually urged to consume more and more in a society dominated by ads and trends, often without contemplating the implications.

The fast fashion business is one of the primary ways that consumption leads to waste. Fast fashion encourages the manufacturing of low-cost, stylish apparel that is swiftly discarded after a few uses. The massive manufacture and disposal of garments generate massive amounts of textile waste and pollution. The fashion sector is currently one of the largest contributors to global garbage, with negative environmental repercussions.

Similarly, frequent updates and fresh releases fuel the electronics business. Consumers are continuously pushed to buy the latest gadgets and equipment, which leads to the disposal of old and obsolete technology. This causes e-waste, a rising environmental concern in which harmful compounds from electronic gadgets seep into the soil and water, causing major health and environmental dangers.

Consumerism contributes to waste by using single-use goods and unnecessary packaging. Our throwaway society promotes the use of plastic water bottles, coffee cups, and takeaway containers, all of which end up in landfills or pollute our seas. Furthermore, many items are packaged in large quantities of plastic, cardboard, and other materials that are frequently non-recyclable or difficult to recycle. This excessive packing contributes to the overall waste produced by consumption.

This fosters a "throwaway" culture in which products that are still working are ignored in favor of the latest versions. This thinking not only causes excessive waste but also promotes a dangerous cycle of constant consumption.

Planned obsolescence exacerbates consumerism's

role in contributing to waste. Many items are purposely intended to have a shorter lifespan, increasing the likelihood that they will break or become obsolete, forcing a replacement. This not only increases trash creation but also encourages excessive consumption.

To address the problem of waste and consumerism, consumers must make conscientious decisions and consider the environmental effect of their purchases. Choosing higher-quality, longer-lasting items can help minimize waste over time. Furthermore, supporting sustainable and ethical firms that stress fair labor standards and utilize eco-friendly materials will help reduce waste.

Furthermore, government restrictions and policies are critical in mitigating the harmful consequences of consumerism on trash. Mandating recycling programs and imposing tougher rules on trash-generating sectors can result in considerable reductions in waste creation. Incentives for recycling and education on the need for trash reduction can also assist shift consumer behavior.

The persistent need to consume, as well as the pressure to keep up with trends and advancements, results in substantial waste. We can, however, reduce waste and promote a more sustainable future by making mindful choices, supporting sustainable products, and campaigning for stronger rules and recycling activities.

Chapter 8. Recycling and Waste Reduction: Sustainable Future Solutions

As our society faces waste management and resource depletion concerns, effective measures for reducing the environmental impact of our consumption patterns can be implemented.

Recycling is a long-term strategy that entails transforming garbage into valuable products. We can conserve natural resources, reduce energy consumption, and reduce pollution connected with the extraction and creation of new materials via recycling. It is critical to promote and support recycling programs that make it simple and convenient for people to recycle their trash. This includes making recycling containers available to the public, educating the public about what can and cannot be recycled, and developing recycling collection and processing facilities.

Waste reduction, also known as waste prevention or source reduction, aims to reduce waste output at its origin. This includes eliminating superfluous packaging, promoting long-lasting and reusable products, and encouraging ethical consumer behavior. By following the concepts of "reduce, reuse, and recycle," we may reduce waste and save resources.

Businesses and industries, in addition to individual activities, play an important role in recycling and trash reduction. They should commit to employing recycled materials, developing goods for durability and recyclability, and establishing take-back programs as part of their sustainable production methods. Businesses may contribute to a circular economy by implementing these practices into their operations and keeping materials in use for as long as feasible.

Technological improvements are very important in recycling and trash reduction. Advanced sorting systems and efficient recycling technologies, for example, can increase the efficacy and efficiency of recycling operations. For example, advances in plastic recycling technology have enabled the recycling of additional types of plastics, hence increasing the circularity of this material. Furthermore, developing technologies such as bioconversion or anaerobic digestion can assist in the conversion of organic waste into useful resources such as biogas or compost.

Additionally, waste minimization can be encouraged by government laws and regulations. Measures such as waste reduction objectives, packaging laws, and expanded producer responsibility programs can be implemented by governments. Governments may encourage positive change and build a culture of sustainability by holding businesses accountable for their influence on trash creation and offering incentives for waste reduction.

Recycling and trash reduction can only be promoted via education and awareness. Individuals may be taught about the environmental implications of garbage and the significance of proper waste management through public campaigns, schools, and community projects. We encourage individuals to make informed decisions and take actions that contribute to a sustainable future by developing a culture of recycling and trash reduction.

Chapter 9. Inspiring Change Through Education and Awareness

Education and awareness are key components in motivating change and ensuring a sustainable future. We can empower people to make informed choices and take action toward a more sustainable and responsible lifestyle by providing folks with knowledge and creating a deeper awareness of environmental challenges.

One of the most important advantages of education and awareness is that they help individuals realize the environmental impact of their activities. Individuals are more likely to adopt ecologically friendly habits and make conscious decisions that reduce their ecological footprint when they understand the repercussions of their actions. Individuals may be more willing to minimize their usage of single-use plastics and opt for reusable alternatives after learning about the harmful consequences of plastic pollution on marine ecosystems.

Education and public awareness are also important in fostering sustainable consumption and waste management. Individuals may become more mindful of their consumption patterns and make attempts to reduce waste output by learning about the ideas of reducing, reusing, and recycling. Furthermore, education may emphasize the need for effective waste segregation, recycling, and the advantages of composting. People are more inclined to adopt these behaviors in their everyday lives if they understand how they contribute to trash reduction and resource conservation.

Furthermore, awareness helps to improve critical thinking abilities and the ability to critically assess environmental information. In an age of disinformation and greenwashing, it is critical to teach people how to distinguish genuine and accurate environmental information. This enables individuals to make well-informed judgments based on scientific data and credible sources, rather than succumbing to deceptive claims or marketing practices.

Education and awareness may also motivate people to take action and mobilize communities. Individuals who work together to understand environmental challenges may lobby for legislative changes, support local efforts, and promote systemic change. Education fosters a sense of environmental citizenship and empowerment, which opens the door to cooperation and collective effect.

Individuals may also become environmental stewards and advocates for sustainability via education and awareness. Individuals may comprehend the need for sustainable development and contribute toward a more equitable and ecologically fair society by learning about the links between environmental, social, and economic systems. They may then share their knowledge and experiences with others, serving as change agents in their communities and driving good behavioral improvements.

Chapter 10. Case Studies in Waste Management: Successes and Failures

Several case studies have offered significant insights into both successful and unsuccessful waste management techniques throughout the years. We may learn from earlier mistakes and create effective solutions to address waste-related concerns more effectively by analyzing these examples.

The trash management technique used by the city of San Francisco, California, is one such effective case study. The city launched a Zero Waste initiative in 2002, to divert 100% recyclable and compostable products from landfill disposal. This program included a variety of methods, such as promoting recycling and composting, encouraging the use of recyclable items, and enforcing tight waste management standards. As a result, San Francisco has one of the greatest garbage diversion rates in the world, at 80%. The importance of strong leadership, clear goals, and community engagement in obtaining good waste management results is highlighted in this case study.

Another remarkable success story comes from the Brazilian city of Curitiba. Faced with limited waste management resources in the 1980s, the city established an innovative system that combined efficient garbage collection with an emphasis on recycling and sustainability. Curitiba set up recycling stations where locals could trade recyclables for food, bus tickets, or coupons for necessities. This encouraged recycling and lowered the quantity of garbage disposed of in landfills. Furthermore, the city constructed a robust public transit system, which decreased trash from private automobiles even more. Curitiba's trash management methodology became a model for sustainable urban development, highlighting the necessity of innovation, community participation, and integrated solutions for garbage management success.

It is crucial to note, however, that not all waste management case studies have been successful. The Love Canal accident in the United States is one well-known example. Love Canal was a Niagara Falls, New York neighborhood that became a dumping place for chemical waste in the 1940s and 1950s. Due to harmful substances that had seeped into the soil and groundwater, the area had major health issues, including birth deformities and malignancies, in the 1970s. The Love Canal tragedy serves as a vivid reminder of the devastation caused by irresponsible garbage disposal, as well as the necessity for stringent rules and monitoring to prevent similar tragedies.

Nairobi, Kenya's main city, is another major failure in trash management. The Dandora Dumpsite in Nairobi has grown to be one of Africa's largest and most poisonous landfills. The temporary facility has been in operation for more than three decades, receiving thousands of tons of rubbish every day. Residents living near the dumpsite are suffering from serious health problems as a result of noxious gasses, tainted water, and the collapse of garbage hills. Despite efforts to solve the problem, such as the installation of a waste-to-energy facility, the Dandora Dumpsite remains a major environmental concern. This case study emphasizes the significance of proactive planning, long-term solutions, and infrastructure investment to reduce garbage accumulation and its negative consequences on communities.

Case studies in waste management give useful insights into applicable and nonapplicable strategies. Examples such as San Francisco and Curitiba highlight the importance of strong leadership, community participation, and integrated techniques to achieve long-term waste management results. On the other hand, incidents such as Love Canal and Dandora Dumpsite serve as a warning of the disastrous effects of irresponsibility, a lack of restrictions, and poor infrastructure.

Policymakers, communities,

and waste management professionals can learn from success stories and avoid past mistakes by studying these case studies, ultimately working toward a cleaner and healthier future. Case studies like San Francisco and Curitiba show the value of proactive planning, community engagement, and integrated approaches. Failures such as Love Canal and the Dandora Dumpsite, on the other hand, demonstrate the effects of irresponsibility, a lack of rules, and poor infrastructure.

Policymakers, communities, and waste management experts may learn from past experiences and work toward more effective waste management strategies by analyzing these case studies.

Chapter 11. The Way Forward:

Creating a Greener and Cleaner Future

As the globe grapples with today's environmental concerns, creating a greener and cleaner future has become critical. Climate change, pollution, and resource depletion are all pressing challenges that must be addressed. Fortunately, there is a growing understanding of the value of sustainable practices and the possibility for good change.The move to renewable energy sources is a critical component in creating a better future. Investing in solar, wind, and geothermal energy may lessen our reliance on fossil fuels while also lowering greenhouse gas emissions. Countries such as Denmark and Iceland have already achieved significant advances in renewable energy adoption, proving that it is feasible to build a vibrant economy while reducing environmental concerns.

In addition to switching to renewable energy, we must reconsider our mobility strategy. The growing popularity of electric cars (EVs) presents a viable approach to reducing carbon emissions from the transportation sector. EVs are becoming more accessible and efficient as battery technology and charging facilities improve. Investing in public transit, bicycle infrastructure, and walkable neighborhoods can also assist to reduce dependency on private automobiles and promote sustainable mobility.

Adopting circular economy ideas is another key part of creating a greener future. This entails moving away from a linear "take-make-waste" approach and toward a circular system in which resources are reused, recycled, or regenerated. Designing goods with recyclability in mind, putting in place effective recycling procedures, and encouraging the use of recycled materials are all critical steps toward establishing a circular economy. Companies such as Patagonia and IKEA have already adopted this strategy, proving that sustainability and profitability can coexist.

Furthermore, waste management procedures must be adjusted to reduce the amount of garbage disposed of in landfills. Implementing successful recycling and composting programs, encouraging trash reduction through education and awareness campaigns, and investing in cutting-edge technologies such as waste-to-energy plants are all ways to divert garbage away from landfills.

A greener and cleaner future also requires the preservation and restoration of ecosystems. The preservation of forests, wetlands, and other natural ecosystems is critical for biodiversity conservation and climate change mitigation. Promoting sustainable agriculture methods, preventing deforestation, and investing in large-scale reforestation programs can all help to sequester carbon and restore the environment.

Education and awareness are critical in creating a greener future. We can develop an attitude of responsible consumption, waste reduction, and conservation by teaching individuals, communities, and future generations about environmental sustainability. Governments, non-profit groups, and educational institutions all play important roles in fostering environmental literacy and enabling people to make sustainable decisions.

Furthermore, policy reforms and international collaboration are required to achieve a greener and cleaner future. Governments must set lofty goals and enact stringent laws to reward sustainable behavior and penalize bad behavior. International treaties, such as the Paris Agreement, provide a framework for collective action and collaboration in the fight against climate change and environmental damage.

To create a greener and cleaner future, all sectors of society must collaborate and work together. Individuals, businesses, governments, and organizations must work together to prioritize sustainability and implement the required adjustments to lessen our environmental effects. We can pave the way for a more sustainable and prosperous future by investing in renewable energy, rethinking transportation, implementing circular economy principles, optimizing waste management, protecting ecosystems, promoting environmental education, and enacting effective policies.

Conclusion

A Shared Vision for a Greener World

We all must work together to create a better world. This vision outlines our goals for protecting and restoring the health of our planet, guiding us toward a more sustainable future for all. A cohesive vision leverages the strength and combined efforts of governments, companies, communities, and individuals to pave the way for the impending environmental revolution.

The realization that our activities today have a direct influence on the well-being and viability of future generations is at the heart of this concept. The urgency of moving to a low-carbon economy is central to this. This necessitates a rapid shift away from reliance on fossil fuels and toward the sustainable creation and usage of renewable energy sources. We can drastically cut greenhouse gas emissions and alleviate the consequences of climate change by pushing clean, carbon-neutral technologies like solar, wind, and geothermal power.

A centered focus on sustainable and circular activities is also critical in reaching a cleaner world. To embrace the concepts of a circular economy, we must prioritize resource efficiency and reuse, reduce waste output, and promote recycling and upcycling. This needs a paradigm change in production and consumption patterns, pushing firms and individuals alike to embrace sustainable practices, decrease carbon footprints, and prioritize natural resource preservation.

The key cornerstones of this united vision are collaboration and cooperation. Environmental challenges transcend national borders, demanding international cooperation to properly solve them. Governments must band together to embrace global sustainability objectives and policies that assist the transition to a cleaner planet. The United Nations Sustainable Development Goals and the Paris Agreement, for example, provide frameworks for coordinating activities and pooling resources in pursuit of sustainability.

This perspective, however, is not confined to governmental actors. Industries have a critical role in influencing change. Innovation and research must be used to produce long-term solutions and practices that minimize pollution and environmental impact across all industries. Businesses must also implement environmentally friendly strategies that incorporate corporate social responsibility and sustainable supplier chains.

Individuals, too, have an indispensable role in achieving a cleaner world. It is essential to raise awareness and empower people with the knowledge and tools to make sustainable choices in their daily lives. Individuals may be educated about the need for environmental conservation through education, outreach initiatives, and public awareness campaigns, which can induce behavior changes that contribute to the goal of a cleaner world. Lastly, without social justice at its center, this cohesive vision is incomplete. We must guarantee that the advantages of a cleaner world are delivered equally, addressing environmental inequities and safeguarding disadvantaged communities from the negative consequences of climate change and pollution. Environmental justice advocates for equitable access to clean air, water, and a healthy environment for all people, regardless of socioeconomic background or geographic location.

Embracing the Responsibility of Stewardship

Stewardship entails caring for, protecting, and managing the Earth and its resources responsibly for current and future generations. It necessitates a paradigm shift in which we see ourselves not as conquerors or consumers of the planet, but as caretakers and custodians with a responsibility to preserve and protect its delicate ecosystems.

Natural resources are finite, and their depletion or degradation can have far-reaching negative consequences, according to the concept of stewardship. It urges us to embrace sustainable methods that encourage responsible resource usage and conservation. Rather than exploiting them for short-term advantage, we should prioritize long-term survival and ecological health.

To accept stewardship responsibility, we must first recognize that our activities have an influence on the environment and that we must reduce negative consequences and increase good ones. This may be accomplished through lowering greenhouse gas emissions, saving water and energy, establishing sustainable agriculture techniques, and maintaining biodiversity, among other things.

Furthermore, stewardship entails acknowledging the interconnectedness of all living beings and ecosystems. It entails realizing that our actions not only have an impact on the natural world but also the well-being and livelihoods of human communities. We can work towards a more equitable and sustainable future for all if we take responsibility for our collective actions.

Accepting the stewardship responsibility necessitates a commitment to education and awareness. We can instill a deep understanding and appreciation for the natural world through education, fostering a sense of connection and empathy for it. We can empower individuals to make informed choices and take purposeful actions that align with the principles of stewardship by raising awareness of environmental issues and their implications.

Stewardship also necessitates collaboration and group action. No single person or entity can address the daunting global challenges we face on its own. Governments, communities, corporations, and people must work together to share information, resources, and best practices. We can collaboratively design and implement effective solutions to protect the earth and promote sustainable development via partnerships and collaboration.

By accepting the stewardship obligation, we not only conserve the environment but also create the groundwork for a more affluent and sustainable future. Stewardship fosters creativity because it forces us to devise novel solutions to complicated environmental problems. It promotes resilience by preparing us to adapt to the changes and difficulties caused by climate change and other environmental crises. Stewardship also fosters social and economic fairness by ensuring that the advantages of a cleaner, more sustainable environment are enjoyed by all.

Appendix

Resources for Taking Action

Numerous crucial resources may enable people and communities to take action when it comes to creating a cleaner planet. These materials provide tools, advice, and support systems that help individuals to make educated decisions and contribute to good environmental change. Let's examine some of these crucial resources for action.

Knowledge and Education: Knowledge is a strong resource for creating change. Access to accurate and up-to-date information on environmental issues and sustainable practices gives individuals the understanding essential to take action. Educational institutions, internet platforms, and community groups play a significant role in disseminating knowledge and encouraging environmental literacy. By encouraging knowledge and creating awareness, learners of all ages may be empowered to make more sustainable choices and advocate for change.

Technology and Innovation: Technological innovations continue to play a significant role in promoting sustainable practices. Tools such as renewable energy technology, energy-efficient appliances, and smart home systems help individuals to lessen their ecological footprint. Additionally, creative solutions in waste management, agriculture, transportation, and manufacturing have the potential to decrease resource consumption and environmental effect. Supporting research and development in sustainable technology leads to a larger array of possibilities for individuals and groups working for a cleaner future.

Policy and Governance: Government rules and regulations offer a framework for influencing sustainable practices and behaviors. Effective policies may incentivize eco-friendly behaviors through tax incentives, subsidies, and laws that support environmentally responsible practices. Additionally, international accords and cooperation, such as the Paris Agreement and the United Nations Framework Convention on Climate Change, contribute to global efforts towards a cleaner planet. Lobbying for improved environmental regulations, interacting with local and national governments, and participating in public consultations are ways individuals may contribute to policy changes that support sustainability.

Community and teamwork: Collective action and teamwork are crucial for establishing enduring change. Participating in environmental organizations, community groups, or sustainability programs allows you to share resources, ideas, and experiences. Engaging with like-minded people develops a feeling of community, which increases efforts to make the world a cleaner place. Collaborative acts, such as neighborhood clean-ups, tree planting projects, and public awareness campaigns, reinforce individual efforts and generate a beneficial ripple effect.

Funding and Investment: Financial resources are essential for organizing action for a cleaner planet. Investing in renewable energy, green infrastructure, and sustainable enterprises speeds up the transition to a low-carbon economy. Individuals and groups working towards environmental sustainability can get money from philanthropic foundations, impact investors, and government grants. Furthermore, sustainable banking and investing choices enable people to connect their financial resources with their ideals.

Personal decisions: Every individual can make everyday decisions that contribute to a cleaner environment. Personal decisions may have a huge influence on the environment, from avoiding trash and choosing sustainable goods to using green transportation and eating a plant-based diet. Everyone has access to resources for action such as conscious consumption, ethical travel, and eco-friendly lifestyle choices.

The above-mentioned resources for action are essential assets that may empower people and communities to contribute to a cleaner world. Knowledge and education, technology and innovation, policy and governance, community and cooperation, finance and investment, and personal decisions are all important factors in creating good environmental change. We can jointly make a huge impact in maintaining and protecting our world for future generations by utilizing these resources and taking action.

Environmental Change Organizations and Initiatives

Numerous groups and projects are fostering good environmental change in the battle against environmental degradation and climate change. These groups, which range from non-governmental organizations (NGOs) to grassroots movements, are at the forefront of advocating for sustainability, raising awareness, and putting real solutions in place. Let's take a deeper look at some of the groups and programs that are working hard to make the world a cleaner, more sustainable place.

Non-Governmental Organizations (NGOs): NGOs such as Greenpeace, WWF, and Friends of the Earth are committed to environmental protection and pushing for sustainable practices. Through campaigns and projects, they perform scientific research, fight for improved environmental regulations, and promote public awareness. These organizations operate on a worldwide scale, cooperating with governments, corporations, and communities to address critical environmental concerns.

UN Environment Programme (UNEP): UNEP is the world's foremost environmental authority inside the United Nations system. It advises and assists governments in developing sustainable policies and practices. To solve critical environmental concerns, UNEP develops international collaboration, manages environmental treaties, and supports the Sustainable Development Goals (SDGs).

The Intergovernmental Panel on Climate Change (IPCC) is a scientific organization founded by the United Nations and the World Meteorological Organization. It gives objective scientific information to policymakers on climate change, its effects, and viable adaptation and mitigation actions. The IPCC reports play an important role in establishing worldwide climate policies and agreements.

The Global Climate Action Summit (GCAS): The Global Climate Action Summit (GCAS) is an effort that brings together governments, corporations, and organizations to highlight climate action and pledges. The summit's goal is to hasten the implementation of the Paris Agreement and inspire more action to combat climate change. The GCAS provides a forum for leaders to discuss best practices, exchange ideas, and cooperate on creative solutions.

The Ellen MacArthur Foundation promotes the circular economy and the transition away from a linear, wasteful paradigm of production and consumption. It collaborates with businesses, governments, and academics to create and promote environmentally friendly methods that eliminate waste, increase resource efficiency, and minimize environmental damage.

Youth-Led Movements: Greta Thunberg's Fridays for Future campaign has garnered worldwide attention and motivated millions of young people to demand immediate action on climate change. Strikes, protests, and educational events are organized by these organizations, elevating the voices of young activists and pushing for aggressive environmental action from governments and companies.

Corporate Sustainability Initiatives: Many businesses are taking steps to decrease their environmental impact and encourage sustainable practices. Companies such as Patagonia, Interface, and IKEA have undertaken ambitious sustainability initiatives such as lowering greenhouse gas emissions, investing in renewable energy, and using circular economy ideas. Their efforts show that firms may be lucrative while still being ecologically responsible.

Community-Based groups: Grassroots groups,

frequently headed by local communities, play an important role in fostering grassroots environmental change. These groups are concerned with specific concerns in their areas, such as preserving local ecosystems, supporting sustainable agriculture, or lobbying for clean energy. They develop a sense of ownership and responsibility for the environment via community participation and education. These groups and projects play a critical role in raising awareness, lobbying for policy reforms, and advancing practical solutions for a cleaner, more sustainable society. Their combined efforts motivate and empower individuals, communities, and governments to take proactive actions to protect our world. We can speed the transition to a more sustainable future for everybody by assisting and partnering with these groups.

Reading Lists and Documentaries

There are various recommended reading materials and videos that give excellent insights and viewpoints to expand our awareness of environmental concerns and encourage action. These resources highlight the importance of the challenges we face and provide ideas and solutions for a more sustainable future. Here are a few prominent suggestions:

"The Sixth Extinction": An Unnatural History" by Elizabeth Kolbert - This Pulitzer Prize-winning book investigates the ongoing mass extinction of species and draws attention to the devastating effects of human activities on biodiversity, serving as a wake-up call to the urgent need for conservation and highlighting the interconnectedness of all life forms on Earth.

"Silent Spring" by Rachel Carson – A classic environmental book, "Silent Spring" is a groundbreaking exploration of the harmful effects of synthetic pesticides, particularly DDT, on ecosystems and human health, inspiring a global environmental movement and leading to DDT bans in several countries.

"Cradle to Cradle": Remaking the Way We Make Things" by Michael Braungart and William McDonough - This book advocates for a move from a linear economy to a circular economy, offering a compelling vision for a sustainable future. It supports the idea of creating items with recyclability in mind and emphasizes the significance of rethinking our production and waste management methods.

**"An Inconvenient Truth"
(2006)** - Directed by Davis
Guggenheim, this
documentary stars former
Vice President Al Gore as he
delivers a riveting and
thorough depiction of
climate change's effects.
The film emphasizes the
importance of the issue and
urges prompt action to
alleviate its consequences.
**"Cowspiracy: The
Sustainability Secret"
(2014)** - Directed by Kip
Andersen and Keegan Kuhn,
this documentary
investigates the
environmental
consequences of animal
husbandry, such as
deforestation, water
pollution, and greenhouse
gas emissions. It
emphasizes the significance
of embracing plant-based
diets and environmentally
friendly farming techniques
to minimize climate change
and safeguard the
ecosystem.

"Chasing Coral" (2017) – Jeff Orlowski's documentary illustrates the disastrous impacts of coral bleaching caused by rising ocean temperatures. It is a call to action to safeguard coral reefs, which are critical ecosystems for marine biodiversity and coastal populations' livelihoods.

"Before the Flood" (2016) – This documentary, directed by Fisher Stevens and produced by Leonardo DiCaprio, follows DiCaprio as he travels the world to investigate the effects of climate change and the measures being done to counteract it. It provides a thorough and fascinating viewpoint on the critical importance of tackling climate change.

These are just a few suggestions; there is a multitude of readings and videos accessible to enlighten and inspire action. Exploring these materials may help us gain a better awareness of environmental issues, drive us to make more sustainable choices, and empower us to help create a greener, cleaner future.

Suggestions for Living More Sustainably

Living more sustainably is becoming increasingly vital as we attempt to lessen our environmental footprint and create a more environmentally friendly future. Here are some suggestions for living more sustainably and making positive changes in your everyday life:

Reduce, reuse, and recycle: the well-known "3 R's" are a good place to start. Reduce your consumption by purchasing only what you require, reusing products wherever feasible, and recycling materials such as paper, plastic, glass, and metal. This contributes to waste reduction and resource conservation.

Conserve energy by turning off lights, appliances, and other electrical devices when they are not in use. Replace incandescent light bulbs with energy-saving LED bulbs. Unplug chargers and other gadgets that utilize power even when they are not in use. Install a programmable thermostat to better manage your home's energy consumption.

Reduce water use by repairing leaks, installing low-flow fixtures, and taking shorter showers. Gather rainwater and use it to water your plants and yard. Run the dishwasher and washing machine just when the loads are full, or change the water level accordingly.

Consume locally, organically, and seasonally as much as possible. Support local farmers, decrease food transportation emissions, and avoid foods that have been excessively pesticide and chemical-treated. Because animal husbandry has a big environmental effect, try integrating more plant-based meals into your diet.

Avoid using single-use plastics: Plastic waste is a big environmental concern. Reusable shopping bags, water bottles, and coffee mugs are preferable. Say no to straws and utensils made of plastic. Look for eco-friendly packaging and items with minimum or biodegradable packaging.

Use conscious transportation: Whenever practical, choose sustainable modes of transportation such as walking, cycling, or taking public transportation. Carpooling or car-sharing can also help to cut greenhouse gas emissions. If you must drive, keep your car in good condition and attempt to combine tasks to reduce trips.

Compost: Start composting instead of tossing organic waste in the garbage. It's an excellent technique to cut trash while also producing nutrient-rich soil for your plant. Composting can save a considerable amount of your home trash from being disposed of in landfills.

Shop with intention: Support companies that value sustainability and ethical practices. Investigate the company you buy from, check for certifications such as Fair Trade and Organic, and pick items created from environmentally friendly components. Consider buying used things wherever feasible to decrease waste and extend product lives.

Plant native species in your garden that require less watering and upkeep to conserve water and safeguard natural resources. To encourage healthy soil, use natural and organic fertilizers. The use of harsh chemicals or pesticides that can affect the environment and wildlife should be avoided.

Educate and inspire people by sharing your expertise and experiences. Encourage your friends, family, and community to embrace environmentally friendly behaviors. You may have a good influence and inspire others to live more sustainably by leading by example and sharing awareness.

It is a journey to live more sustainably, and every tiny step matters. Remember, it's not about being flawless, but about making conscientious decisions that support a greener, more sustainable lifestyle. By following these suggestions, you may help to make the world a healthier and more sustainable place for future generations.